What's In A Name?

What's In A Name?

Turner Stimpson

T·U·R·N·I·P
TRUST · UNDERSTANDING · RESPECT · NURTURED · INNER · PEACE

Warren Publishing, Inc.

ISBN 1-886057-73-7

Manufactured in the United States of America
First Edition
19809 North Cove Road
Cornelius, North Carolina 28031
www.warrenpublishing.net

Dedication

For all those special people, who have touched my life since I answered God's knock in 1990, I thank you. I also thank many of you for being the real stars in our documentary, "Love Spoken Here: A Day in the Life of Turnip, Approaching Alzheimer's with Hope and Joy." –filmed August 22, 2003 and shown January 21, 2004 on PBS; but, most importantly, I thank you for giving me purpose and meaning in my life through your amazing love, courage, and sense of humor.

And lastly, I thank my precious wife, Mickey M. Stimpson, who through God's blessings and almost 35 years of marriage, has taught me the real proof of being a good teacher-keep it simple, be consistent and show love.

And, since my wife's diagnosis of cancer on January 23, 2004, she has taught me even more. I know I married a miraculous lady, who has shown me joy, hope, and love.. Thanks be to God and "My Boomer."

Turner "Turnip" Stimpson

About the Author

What's In A Name is the third book that Turner Stimpson has authored. He continues to work as the Resident Care and Transportation Coordinator of The Pines at Davidson, a life care community in Davidson, North Carolina.

The year 2004 marked many milestones and highlights in Turner's career. As keynote speaker, he has traveled across the United States speaking out against the prevailing negative image of Alzheimer's, all the while, changing the "face" of Alzheimer's.

Turner continues to touch lives by reaching beyond the fear of Alzheimer's and spreading his message of joy and hope.

He and his lovely wife, Mickey, reside in Statesville, North Carolina. Turner would love to hear from you and encourages you to contact him at his web site: *theTurnipApproach.com*.

What's In A Name?
Foreword

"Love received or given in any circumstance or condition is a precious thing."
(*What's In A Name?* p. 39)

Once again, Turner "Turnip" Stimpson has gifted the community of those acquainted with Alzheimer's disease with a wonderful book. This book has a universal dimension to it. Turner encourages the reader to reflect on the meaning of love and the power of memory in his/her life. He gently reveals a remarkable paradox: memory can be created in the very moment of forgetting. Turner reminds us that having "visions of the heart" is central to meaningful life.

In *What's In A Name?*, Turner (with his trademark *innocent vulnerability*) shares his love-filled memories with us of persons who have touched his life in an *everlasting* way. He confides in us, allowing us to enter his world of care giving for persons with dementia. It is as though we have walked into a theater and have been given "Turnip spectacles" through which to view the world of aging and dementia. We see how "Turnip" *remembers persons with dementia into the present through re-naming them in a way that speaks their personhood into being*. We demonstrates the significance of a name by gifting his beloved care receivers with nicknames that connect to their spirit.

In this latest volume, Turner reminds us that the Turnip Approach is about relationship. As I read through *What's In A Name?*, I experienced tears, laughter, and delight; I recalled the things in life that matter the most to everyone. Turner suggests that simplicity is essential if we are to feel the "joy and hope that comes from two people sharing love and a good time together."

He reminds us that the encounters we often think are without meaning or merit are the very encounters that have the capacity for revealing the profound in the ordinary. In this way, *What's In A Name?* offers a dimension of universality to all who read it for it reminds us to celebrate the moments of "memory making" that grace our lives each and every day if we are willing to receive love and to share life with another.

What's In A Name? is a wonderful book that honors the lives of persons with dementia through the sharing of their life giving "memories in the making." Turner honors their stories, acknowledging that the lives of persons with dementia are continuing to create important, meaningful stories even in the midst of weakening conditions. In *What's In A Name?*, Turner encourages us to allow God to grace us with the gift of continuing to love others no matter "what condition one's condition is in." Thank you, Turner, for gifting us with a book that is infused with the loving spirit of God that graces us all for the living and giving of our days!

Rev. Betsy Haas Faughn, M. Div., MSW, LCSW
Charlotte, North Carolina

What's in a Name?

What's in a name? It's funny what you remember about a person. Sometimes what you remember most vividly can seem so trivial. So ordinary. Like a ripple on life's little pond. Other times what you remember is the very thing you know you'd always remember. The name you have written on your heart.

As you read "What's In A Name," I pray that you will just get aboard on a journey played out by "Real" leading actors. It is my hope the journey will take you places in which you feel joy, love, and an *Inner Peace* that you never felt before. Perhaps some of you will even come to realize what your true gifts are—the fact that you too have the gift of love. All of a sudden you want to be a miracle for these special people.

In any event, there's joy, hope, and yes, love out there for these special people, if we will just be "a vehicle of love." I promise, you will find an *Inner Peace* that you have never felt before. And, together we will change the face of ALZHEIMER'S. The outlook will be bright because there is love.

For those of you who do not know me, in my first life, I was a 3rd generation hosiery manufacturer of a family owned business. I have many wonderful memories of those days. My job allowed me to travel to New York where the Mill's selling agency was located in the Empire State Building. It was in my travels to NY that I saw the Yankees play, and I acquired some awesome autographs. My wife used to model the new trends in panty hose, even the neon colors. Much to my wife's chagrin, I even stretched the hosiery on mannequins when we went shopping. I was just checking out the competition.

These moments I remember, but I don't have these moments anymore. One, because my wife won't let me, but the most important reason is God. He wants me to be a part of moments much more important than our economy. It is these moments that have brought us together.

When I say, "God has a sense of humor," I truly mean this. From the factory floor to care giving is quite a transformation. My wife said to me, "Honey, I found you in the Bible. It is 1 Corinthians 1:26-29." Curious, I looked it up. Paul writes, "But God chose what is foolish in the world to confound the wise." Well, that's me, the last and the least! But here I am, about to tell about care giving moments, and "What's in A Name?"

"What **is** in a name?" A name can refer to people, places, and events. Take a moment to reflect on certain people, places, and events in your past that have had an everlasting influence on your journey through life. Do you remember any special people? What about places? And, what about events? I believe each one of you were able to name special people, places, and events—so, what's in a name? A personal name, I believe is our very essence. A name is up close and personal and can be a reflection of our worth in the eyes of others. A name can reflect on your ancestry. A name can give one a certain amount of self-esteem and more importantly, meaning in one's life. We all yearn for meaning in our lives, so what about me?

Like each of you, I have also been influenced by certain people, places, and events. And, like you, there are some that literally changed my whole being. The first was the meeting of my wife, which has culminated in our marriage of nearly 35 years. What an exchange of meeting and sharing of our names, upon our first introduction. My wife's birth name is Mickey Michael, and of course, my name is Turner Stimpson. At first glance, you recognize she has two first names, (both boys names) and I have two last names, (family names). My wife is the daughter of a golf pro. Her name came from the desire of a golf family wanting a son, while my name came from the Turner and Stimpson family. While growing up, my wife's name gave her a certain amount of confidence and self-esteem. She was cute (and still is) and the name was cute and had a ring to it, like Mickey Mantle. In my name, I not only represented two families, but I also represented a place, Turnersburg. My great grandmother's brother, L. Dent Turner, was Lieutenant Governor of North Carolina. Whereas, upon meeting me for the first time, my wife thought my name was Stimpson Turner. My mother had said to me growing up that I liked baseball so much that I would probably marry someone named Mickey, like Mickey Mantle—how uncanny! I know everything was meant to be.

The second major event came, as I became "TURNIP." By the slip of the tongue of Miss Mourne, a dementia patient in my charge, I became "TURNIP." She was calling out to me. "TURNIP, I want to be with "TURNIP." I knew then that I was making a difference in someone's life. I knew that God had given me a very large heart, along with it the gift of love. It was time to recognize this precious gift and use it. Long before I became TURNIP, I believed if I could help each person in my charge obtain *inner peace,* then I would have reached one of my objectives. It was also my hope that if I made each resident feel safe, secure and at the same time special, my goal would be accomplished; however, I believed God wanted me to do more for these special people. This thought brings to recollection my hosiery days, and in particular, an article I wrote for a business magazine. The article was titled, "God Loves The Small Business, Too." In this article, I compared the small business or mill to a small creature of God's Kingdom. We both can die, if we don't use the gifts that God has given each of us to survive. However, I don't believe God wants these cognitive impaired people to just survive. He wants their lives to have meaning and purpose, thus making their names of essence in the place that really counts—their hearts. What's in a name? And, how can I help to give these special people's lives purpose?

After becoming "TURNIP," one day I was doodling in a staff meeting with the letters which make up the word "TURNIP." Miraculously, an acronym came about:

T + Trust
U + Understanding
R + Respect
N + Nurtured =
I + Inner
P + Peace

Was the nickname chance? Or the acronym, which followed? No, I believe everything and everyone has a special purpose. The acronym became a successful model to use to gain trust and love of a dementia patient. As demonstrated in "Octopus" from the book written by C. M. Stimpson, TURNIP, Why Are We Here?, a dementia patient fearful of the bath is not afraid anymore. "Suddenly, then, the "man in the white coat" becomes TURNIP—someone who loves me—someone who takes care of me—someone who will not wheel me to my doom—someone who will protect me from the strangeness of this event—someone who will see me through—someone to hold my hand in the darkness... And an octopus becomes an odd looking chair—and it's venom, my bath water."

Since I've now gained trust in the dementia patient, it is time to give him a feeling of purpose in his life. How will I do this? What about a nickname? I've used nicknames for many years, especially with my employees in the hosiery business. I give credit to a psychology professor in college, who believed if nicknames were used appropriately they could be a very positive thing. Nicknames come about after a thorough study of an individual's personality. So call your charge by a nickname. It will give him/her self-esteem. Make the nickname a reflection of this individual person. First, it will cue them in on their past, but most importantly, it will give purpose to their life. For example, there is a lady I call " Miss Chesterfield." I call her this because she came from Chesterfield and she was the beauty queen. You ought to see her light up when I call her "Miss Chesterfield." I know she feels special and has meaning in her life. You can see all of this in her eyes. Her nickname was an easy one; however, others are more difficult to come up with. That's the case with the one I'm about to tell you. During the process of trying to find a perfect fit, this special lady expressed repeatedly her desire to have a nickname and, as time lapsed, she said, "You won't come up with a nickname for me?" Her desire for a nickname made the task even more challenging. I perceived she felt left out because I did not have a nickname for her. It made me realize, though, how important nicknames really are. If they were not so important, why would she want one?

Coming up with a nickname for this amazing lady probably has given me more satisfaction than anything; however, it's not just the fact of coming up with the nickname, but what the nickname did for our relationship. Let me tell you about this lady. She is a retired schoolteacher having taught the 5th grade for many years in North Carolina. She has always been exceedingly private and I always respected her wishes.

As her health weakened, she became closer to me—not affectionate, but closer. It's amazing what happened after I coined her "My Favorite Keeper." From that moment she became closer and closer to me. She showed affection. We bonded. The nickname was the answer. I had picked a name perfect for her.

On outings, I would let her be boss. I'd ask her about the time and when to go home and she loved it. Can't you just picture her in the 5th grade leading class and instructing her students. Thanks to "My Favorite Keeper," I am instructed on a daily basis from a lady who now loves me and wants me to do right and she is and always will be "My Favorite Keeper."

As mentioned earlier, sometimes I have an easy time coming up with a perfect nickname for that special person, like "Miss Chesterfield," while other times are more difficult, like "My Favorite Keeper." It is now time to relax and get on board for a journey of joy and hope. Although some nicknames were easy for me and some were hard and others are just names, they all blessed me more than words can ever express. Sit back and enjoy the ride "a mission of love"!

"My Queen Call"

When I stop to reflect on this special lady, my first thought is of a lady, who happened to become a queen, "My Queen Call." Happened is probably not the right word to use s _ _ _ happens (get the picture) but not becoming a queen. Like angels, which have to be found, I believe God enabled me to find "My Queen Call," or perhaps we found each other. Anyway, I believe we gave purpose to each other's lives.

"My Queen Call" was from Piedmont, North Carolina where she taught school in her earlier years. As mentioned in our book "Love Spoken Here," it is pretty easy to pick out the teachers at The Pines. They all have the mode of instruction when asking me to do things for them. They instruct me! “My Queen Call” did this too, but what a sense of humor. Many of the Southern sayings and slang that this ole boy uses was part of her life too. This made for a very special and unique bond. She also liked to watch baseball on T.V. Many times I would stay at night and watch the Braves with her. She loved this and I did too. We pretty much watched games together on a regular basis, especially after her husband died.

Although we got closer and closer after her husband’s death, like “My Favorite Author” and “Queen B,” I believe, like with so many residents, our greatest joys were on outings together. Residents loved to take a ride. And, through God’s help, even medical appointments became an opportunity to experience the serenity of this world and most importantly, feel the joy and hope that comes from two people sharing love and a good time together. Things should be simple. It should be about relationships and love. This was the case with “My Queen Call” and me. What a time we always had together. What laughs and fun! My only regret is that I never had a Queen sign installed in the little ambulance that we traveled in together. I had promised her that one day we would have that sign and we would raise the sign and pass all the traffic in Charlotte, as if she was the Queen of England. One day, I’ll get that sign because I believe I’ll find more Queens in my life, if only I will leave my heart open and let love have a chance to flow through God’s blessings. If I will only receive, but first I am thankful for “My Queen Call.” She was very special to me and gave me a reason to call out for more Queens—thanks, “My Queen Call”—I will always love you!

"The Lady From Bristol"

What a lady! Like many of our stories, my fondest memories with "The Lady from Bristol" came while I was performing Private Nursing. As mentioned many times, I believe Private Nursing is the best type of nursing. In this nursing, one has the opportunity to bond with a patient and you really get to know each other. As a result, you have created together an environment conducive for joy, hope, and love. This was the case with this special lady and me.

Although we had many times together, I remember taking her to the little Davidson public library. She really loved to read books, but with each excursion I wondered if we were checking out our last book or not. Davidson folks will remember the little library. Simply wall-to-wall people and books were in some cramped quarters. Speaking of "no room in the Inn," this made it look like a farce. Just picture a precious, little lady with a cane and grasping my pants as if she didn't ever want to let go and my arms full of books. We were an accident about to happen... really! But, through it all, there was a bond of love that was tighter than the grip she had on my pants. There was hope, joy, and yes, love, and I knew this was a wonderful world, even in the library. Come to think of it, that is where I met my wife (not this library, of course) but a library. Sometimes, just as you cannot tell a book by the cover, sometimes the words are not what's important in the book. It may just be the experience it leads you to; and just sometimes, the experience might turn into love.

Sometimes love can be funny too! That's the case with a vivid experience between this lady and me. This experience happened at Harris Teeter's grocery store in Cornelius. You guessed it, we were shopping and, you probably also guessed, as in the library she was holding onto my Dockers. We together were in search for a suitable Wheaties box, however, all of the boxes were gigantic, just as all things seem to be today. It was at this point that this special lady's sense of humor arose to the front. She said, "Turner, I won't be able to eat that box of cereal in a lifetime, but if it's toilet paper, get it." What a memory. What a lady. As time lingered on and as she weakened, we became closer and closer and shared many more memories together. This lady will always be in my heart and, yes, I'll always remember the two stories I just told. But most important, I will never forget the love that God gave to us just for the asking. And, yes, I wonder every now and then if she's got my book in heaven. I believe she does. If so, we both will have each other's manuscript. She gave me a book that is in my heart forever!

"Miss Book Circle"

I know you must be thinking, why on earth would "TURNIP" give somebody a nickname like this? Well, the nickname really fits. Like "The Lady from Bristol, " this special lady loved books too. And, like the "Lady from Bristol," she was weakening and was needing the love and care that I believe God put me here to give. And, like many people, including myself, this special lady was stubborn. She needed help, a lot of help, but she didn't think so. Really deep down I believe she knew she needed assistance, however, like many people, her pride prevented her from saying "uncle." As her health continued to weaken, it became apparent something had to be done. I became the reluctant answer. Let me say, I was not reluctant—she was. The idea was for me to be "Miss Book

Circle's" escort. After agonizing for sure, probably for weeks, she finally decided that the idea wasn't so bad after all. Little did I know, that I would become "escort personified" and personified is putting it mildly! I know the meaning of being an escort was never the same again, at least not for me!

Although "Miss Book Circle's" physical and mental capacities had weakened greatly and her memory had gone "out to lunch," she was still pretty sharp. Her sharpness required me to change my whole calendar to accommodate. And, accommodate I did. Let me say, if you Davidson residents have not figured out who "Miss Book Circle" is by now, she is from Davidson. She not only was from Davidson, I believe she was Davidson and knew everybody, which I found out the hard way (literally) at a retirement reception. As mentioned earlier, I became her all-purpose escort. Well, the fact that she knew everybody in Davidson, made her want to take part in every event. We were busy going to Sunday school functions and parties, weddings, receptions, and anything else that she found out about that was going on in this little town. Now to the subject, my memory that will linger the most will be the time I was escorting her to the retirement reception for a beloved religion professor at Davidson College, who happens to be living at The Pines now. Just picture her pushing a cart with a little basket on it and this escort (me) following behind trying to divide the traffic of people and hopefully keep her afloat. As she stopped to talk to each person (and she knew them all) as she pushed her cart, she always had a hand full and mouth full of hors d'oeuvres. At this time, the final count was not in, but I've never seen somebody in her condition being able to talk, eat, drink, and be merry while pushing a cart. I believe God was making this all possible.

I did mention a count, didn't I? Before we go to the count, let me say how amazing it was for me to witness all she was doing. This was quite a feat for me to view. After all, it seemed like it took a lifetime for this ole boy to even learn to tie my shoes and now when I think how long it took before I could e-mail. Amazing lady! The story came to its conclusion as I helped her into the car and buckled her seat belt. Just then, all of a sudden, I felt something stick me hard in the leg—boy did that hurt! She said, "What's happening, Turner?" As I reached into my suit pocket, I realized what the object was that was sticking me—Hors d'oeuvre sticks. Looking into my pocket and gathering the sticks, I began to count. To my surprise, I had 17 sticks, so I must have been eating too. The next thing I knew she exclaimed, "Hell, that's nothing, Turner." She then proceeded to take her sticks out of her pocketbook. To my amazement, she had 29 sticks—I'm glad we didn't save the glasses too!

"Pretty Lib"

What a pretty lady! "Pretty Lib" was very special to me and pretty too! My first memory of this special lady came when she first moved to The Pines and it became apparent to me that maybe her memory had already gone "out to lunch." She was in Independent Living and she carried a little note pad where she was continually writing notes of things, names, and places. I knew she needed help—don't we all? It was through our earlier times together that I began to see the real beauty in this special lady. As I've mentioned many times, Confucius said, "Beauty—Everything has beauty but not everyone sees it." I could really see beauty in this lady. She was elegant and very attractive. You could see beauty through the sparkle in her eyes. The greatest beauty perhaps could not be seen but came from her heart. Just as Helen Keller said, "The best and most beautiful things in the world cannot be seen, nor touched . . . but are felt in the heart." That was the way it was with "Pretty Lib."

As time passed on and this special lady weakened, we got closer and closer. I can still see her light up when I called her "Pretty Lib." I remember all of the outings together and medical appointments and bringing her back and forth from the hospital. But importantly, I remember her spirit and beauty and she was still like a blessing of fresh air. She was just precious, and she gave to me more than I could ever give back to her. She humbled me and made me realize what the Turnip Approach is and should be. It's about relationships. It's about joy, hope, and yes, love. Through her blessings to me through God, I had the gift of *inner peace*. Thanks, "Pretty Lib," I'll never forget you or your love or beauty—that is "Pretty Lib"—I will always love you!

"Frenchie"

When you think of the word "Frenchie," what do you think of? It's my guess that you thought it is a nickname for a French girl. In my first life, my first thought would be "Frenchie" from the movie "Grease." Speaking of "Grease," the play is coming to Charlotte and I'll be taking the residents from The Pines to the play. I'm excited—I just love the play; but each time I think about "Grease," I can't help thinking about Olivia Newton-John. She wasn't "Frenchie," but was the star and did a whole lot for me emotionally or I should say just tore my heart and everything else up! I even got up at 4:00 in the morning to get tickets at the Old Charlotte Coliseum for her only NC appearance ever. I can still remember "Let's Get Physical" and "I Honestly Love You." I think it's time for me to stop rambling and stop with "I Honestly Love You" and get to the story, which happens also to be about love.

I suppose by now, you perhaps by the process of elimination have come to the conclusion that this is a different "Frenchie." The "Frenchie" I'm getting ready to tell you about was not in "Grease" or in my first life, but she certainly has been in my second life and I've been blessed.

Like many nicknames, I spend much time and deliberation before coming up with just the right one for each of these special people. Some are easier than others. This was an easy one, but it seemed to be perfect for this special lady. Like others, the nickname seemed to give purpose to her life and mine. It became the spark that brought us closer and closer. It also created an environment conducive for sharing love and good times together. The nickname bonded us and remained until the end of her life.

"Frenchie" was dubbed her nickname while in Independent Living. It came about from both of us having a love for French Onion Soup, which has always been my favorite soup since tasting it at the Ole Ranch House Restaurant in Chapel Hill, growing up. Well, it's her favorite soup. Both of us also loved to eat at Honey Baked Ham, which, at times, had French Onion Soup on the menu, to our delight.

As this special lady weakened and found herself in Health Care, "Frenchie" and I continued to get closer and closer. Although her short- term memory had really gone "out to lunch," it never prevented us from going "out to lunch," and many times we found ourselves at Honey Baked Ham and enjoyed French Onion Soup. The last time we shared it together came the day before she died. Like the others, you guessed it—we had French Onion Soup. This time we shared joy and love, and, yes, soup at The Little Kitchen Restaurant in Mooresville. Thanks "Frenchie," and I know every time I eat French Onion Soup, I will think of you and think of how much love we shared, not to mention soup!

"Hot Rod Mama"

I must say the nickname coined for this special lady probably has caused more looks of double takes than any nickname. Many of those double takes were directed at me—how crazy! I tell people that I am too blessed to be stressed. You can probably imagine that I also tell them that I am too crazy to be stressed. I believe this to be true, but I am very thankful for the gift of love that I believe God gave me. If I just keep loving, even though I'm human and my heart can hurt too, things seem to always work. It is that faith that is my foundation and keeps me going. As long as there is possibility, we'll keep loving and searching for giving one another hope and joy and perhaps one day we will have *inner peace* everlasting! It seems I got off the subject again; however, I believe love should be a part of everything; and, I might add, love was a part of "Hot Rod Mama"!

Speaking of "Hot Rod Mama," her nickname ranked right up there with "Number 10"; however, her nickname was just perfect for this special lady.

"Hot Rod Mama" grew up in Indiana on a farm. Like many people from Indiana, she was proud of her state. She loved sports and she was even a good athlete. She played basketball in college where she met her husband, who also played basketball, as well as baseball. The couple graduated from the University of Indiana and were naturally extremely proud of their rich basketball tradition. While in Independent Living, as well as in her weakened condition, we had quite a number of interesting conversations regarding the basketball powers of UNC and Indiana and Dean Smith and Bobby Knight. We had a wonderful time together. You are probably thinking that you still do not know where the nickname came from. Well, it's time to tell you. "Hot Rod Mama," as mentioned earlier, was a good athlete and she wanted to do the same sports that a man did, so when her husband took up bike riding or motorcycle riding, she did too. She shared her pictures of those days with me. She looked so happy on that motorcycle. Quite a picture to write home about, wearing the helmet and all—quite a picture!

As she weakened and her short-term memory got shorter, her past, like many of these special people, became more important to her. She remembered so many interesting events in her life that I was blessed that she shared them with me. Some of these events were involving a motorcycle. I really had the fear that we would be riding a motorcycle together. Wouldn't that be an event? If you had the chance to read our first book, I wasn't real good at maneuvering the electric cart in Food Lion. The store was in great danger. I can't imagine how dangerous it would be to ride double with "Hot Rod Mama." It was my prayer, if that was the case, she would be operating the machine and not me!

Thanks, "Hot Rod Mama," for being such a good sport. Love does come in many different forms and takes shape differently, but there is love, and that means all the difference!

"Miss Chesterfield"

Yes, "Miss Chesterfield" is a special lady that I've mentioned many times. Matter of fact, "Miss Chesterfield" was one of the special stars in our book "Love Spoken Here."

"Miss Chesterfield" was one of the easiest nicknames to come up with. After all, she was from Chesterfield and she was the beauty queen. "Miss Chesterfield," I believe, had purpose and meaning in her life until the end. Just the sound of "Miss Chesterfield" lit her up. Her eyes just sparkled. I believe the nickname led her into her past and you know, she was really a beautiful lady, even as she weakened and her mind went "out to lunch." Once a lady, always a lady—that was "Miss Chesterfield."

My first memories of "Miss Chesterfield" came when she was in Independent Living. She loved plays, concerts, and any kind of outing; and she was so elegant. She loved dressing up, and she had wonderful taste in clothes. I know, by now, you are laughing at me. What does TURNIP know about taste in women's clothes? I'd really surprise you. If you haven't heard in my first life, I was a third generation hosiery manufacturer of a family-owned business (panty hose), so I knew women's clothes and after all I've already told you, I might as well admit that I love to shop. On occasions, I've even picked out outfits for our lovely ladies from The Pines at Tanner's and South Park, so when I say I know good taste, I do. Well, "Miss Chesterfield" was beautiful and loved to go places. Like many of our residents, I continued to take these special people to events even after they were in a weakened state and resided in Health Care. "Miss Chesterfield" was one of these special people that continued to go with me at night and bless all of us with her beauty and elegance.

As just mentioned, our last trips together to the theater will remain in my mind and how much fun she still had, even though she was in a weakened condition: however, the memory that I will never forget happened on one of our Health Care Thursday outings on the bus. There's some unusual humor in this story, but what insight!

This outing occurred during the period of time that the new hospital was being built in Mooresville. We had traveled along the road around Lake Norman and were heading back home. As we approached the site where the hospital was being built, I pointed it out to the residents. As we passed by the hospital and within rock throwing distance we came upon a historic church and cemetery. As we drove closer, there was a sign with a small summary of the church and cemetery's history; and no sooner than I had read the sign, I heard coming from the back of the bus through the voice of an amazing lady, "Miss Chesterfield," "Oh, how convenient." What insight! What a movie that could be made! I can just picture someone dying in the hospital and someone opening the window and the body landing squarely on the ground—what a savings!

Thanks, "Miss Chesterfield" for the story and for giving me a beauty queen to love.

"Two Queens w/King Names"

The next special people are not one, but two queens. The nickname, as with each one, came about very easily and almost gives away their real last names. Both were queens and both were extremely smart ladies; even when their health weakened and dementia set in, they both still amazed me with their intelligence. I truly believe if we are able to create an environment built on trust and love, things can happen. It makes it possible for an individual to still be able to show their smarts. This was the case with both of these ladies.

Both ladies, I know, had meaning and purpose in their lives, and they both loved their nicknames. After all, who wouldn't like to be called a "Queen." One was from the South and one was from the North, but both were very special to me. One loved to eat spaghetti, while the other queen loved peppermint ice cream, which I dearly love. Thanks to both Queens w/King names for being a part of my life. I only wish that some of your intelligence would have rubbed off on me!

Mr. Bronson

When I think of Mr. Bronson, I immediately think of the Fiddler. Here's the story.

Every once in awhile in our own lives, we see something amazing and out of the ordinary. The next story falls in that category for sure. Sometimes that extraordinary event occurs more than once in your life. Something that you never dreamed of seeing, now you have seen more than once; however, the first time will be the one you always remember. About 3 years ago, Mr. Bronson and I were returning from a doctor's appointment when suddenly we looked to the side of the road and there he was—The Fiddler. Yes, a man on the side of the road sitting on a stool was fiddling profusely. We could not believe our own eyes! I pulled off the side of the road to get a better look. As I strained my neck out of the window to see if I was really seeing a fiddler, my good friend kept rolling his eyes back and forth wondering what he just saw. Could it really be a fiddler? It is still hard for me to believe what we saw. If Charles Kuralt were still living, this would be a great person to interview. What a day!

Sometimes in life we have certain events that occur in relationships that later become "The Flagship" for that relationship. This was the case with Mr. Bronson and me. It was our moment.

Mr. Bronson is a very special man. He is very kind and is a gentleman. His health, however, has declined recently. He has had a number of mini strokes recently and his dementia is more present but he thinks of the trip we first saw The Fiddler often.

After seeing The Fiddler for the first time, Mr. Bronson told his daughter of our viewing of the fiddler; and she later joked to her father's friends and with us that Turner and her father had been drinking—they had to be if they saw a fiddler on the side of the road—huh?

As done before, from time to time, I allow guests to be a part of our Thursday Healthcare outings. Many times family members ride with us. I think this does wonders for residents as well as their family members. We all have a wonderful time—everyone likes to take a ride. Mr. Bronson's daughter has been aboard on occasions; and each of the times we have headed to the residence of the fiddler hoping he would provide us with excitement and amazement. Each time he was not there when Mr. Bronson's daughter was on the bus; so the drinking theory stayed in place. But, finally, about a month ago, we headed for Concord to see the fiddler and there he was fiddling, fiddling, and fiddling to the delight of Mr. Bronson and at last his daughter saw the fiddler too. It wasn't the last time Mr. Bronson and I saw the fiddler. This special memory will always be in our hearts and I know

Mr. Bronson will always be ready to go and see the fiddler.

"The Pride of Greensboro"

"The Pride of Greensboro," like Mr. Bronson, was another example of a true gentleman. In the 21st Century a true gentleman is a rare thing to find. "The Pride of Greensboro" was a true gentleman and very special.

Although he was in very poor physical condition and his life became one full of strokes and dementia, he remained solid as a rock. He really was the pride of Greensboro. All residents who knew him, had to be extremely proud of him. I will always remember him laughing and having a special twinkle in his eyes. He was delightful and very thoughtful. He remained very appreciative, even in his worse condition. What a blessing! I believe we learn more about a person in a weakened condition than in their better days. We learned so much from "The Pride of Greensboro." Through it all, he was still a gentleman and he remained strong. I've always believed that one can be strong and at the same time gentle. What traits to have. Just as we need to use our God- given gifts, I believe these special people need an environment that is conducive for joy, hope, and yes, love. This will allow them to just be themselves and together we both will have purpose and meaning in our lives; and *Inner Peace*—thanks to "The Pride of Greensboro" and the beloved gentleman!

"Good Cuz"

If "Good Cuz" sounds familiar to you, perhaps you read C.M. Stimpson's and my first book, "TURNIP,

Why Are We Here?" "Good Cuz" brought us the story of "Hotel California." He definitely lived the good life and took advantage of his nice surroundings. If you remember, "Hotel California" was a large double room and "Good Cuz" had two of everything—beds, chester drawers, lamps, T.V.'s, etc. You get the picture. Although this story will be one that I'll never forget, I have another story that will also be in my memory bank forever.

The memory came about at Rocky River Presbyterian Church's Annual Reunion. The cast not only included "Good Cuz," but his cousin "Mr. J" of grape juice and Godzilla fame. Some of you might remember "Mr. J" from the book "TURNIP, Why Are We Here?" I took both special people to this event to their delight, not to mention, their children. During this period of time, "Good Cuz" was getting around real well, after all, at the time, his residence was "Hotel California"; however, his cousin "Mr. J" 's health had declined greatly and he was in a wheelchair and had to be fed. Like many other times and, in particular, when performing private nursing, I've gone without eating. I'm always thinking of who I'm taking care of first. This was the case at Rocky River. "Good Cuz" was having a ball and eating very well, while I spent the majority of my time taking care of his cousin "Mr. J," who was also enjoying his afternoon, even though he had to be fed. After everybody in my charge was in good shape, I began to eat starting with fried chicken, which I dearly love. As in the past, "Good Cuz" was taking everything in and I suppose I was really hungry and maybe I was eating faster than normal; but anyway, "Good Cuz" never forgot me eating chicken. Every family night dinner from Healthcare that we had from then on, "Good Cuz" told everyone how TURNIP could really eat chicken. I do like chicken but I must have liked it even more in the eyes of "Good Cuz." Chicken became a memory for "Good Cuz" but he never forgot the wonderful time we had that Sunday afternoon at Rocky River. Thanks, "Good Cuz" for everything and "Hotel California" too!

"Mr. G."

It's amazing sometimes in life how the world in which we live seems to be smaller. That's the case with "Mr. G." and me. Like many of the residents at The Pines, we have a connection from out of the past. Many times that connection was from Statesville. "Mr. G." and I did business together for many years in our first life—my life as a hosiery manufacturer. Matter of fact, "Mr. G." did business with my father and grandfather earlier; and he had known me since I was a child.

Upon seeing each other in my second life (at The Pines) for the first time, neither one of us knew each other. We both looked at each other like we should know each other, but to no avail. Then suddenly one day as "Mr. G." approached me in the hall, he hollered out, "Turner Stimpson. . . . Stimpson Hosiery Mills, Inc." At last, we knew the connection. "Mr. G." was an insurance representative and our mill had our insurance with him, all the way back to my grandfather. It's funny how we can be so close to someone, but as time elapses and we find people in a different environment, we don't even recognize the person. However, this did not last long. Before long, we were talking our heads off and remembering all of our experiences in business. "Once a friend, always a friend." That was the case with Mr. G." and me. The bond was rekindled and we were blessed by being in each other's company.

As time marched on and "Mr. G.'s" health and memory were in a weakened state, the bond that was built long ago never left. We got closer and closer. "Mr. G." always had a good sense of humor, which he carried with him to the delight of the residents and me. He still had his love for flowers and loved to plant. His green thumb never left him either. Even with his failing health and dementia, I believe he still had meaning and purpose in his life. It's important that we help to create an environment that is conducive for joy, hope, and love. This environment will make it always possible for these special people to continue to be what God created them to be. I pray we will always be able to create an environment where love and *Inner Peace* is possible!

Although there are many memories I'll always have when thinking about "Mr. G." his humor will be most remembered and one thing, in particular. Each time I returned with him from a medical appointment, the barbershop, getting ice cream or flowers, while in the car I came around his side to unbuckle his seat belt, he would always say, "Untie me Villain." I'll always remember that. Thanks, "Mr. G." for coming into both lives—that as a hosiery manufacturer and later, as TURNIP!

"DR. P"

What a mind! When I stop to reflect on "Dr. P," my first thought is of his intelligence. Although he had been a Religion Professor, his knowledge did not stop there. He was so versed on every subject. He could carry on a conversation with anybody and on any subject, from sports to religion to history to politics—he knew them all! The thing that was great about him was the fact; that even though he knew a great deal, he was always very humble. He also had a sense of humor, which everyone loved, including myself.

As I've mentioned many times, one needs a conversation piece to help build a bond with an individual. "Dr. P" and I, like many of the residents at The Pines, had that conversation piece. The piece was my funny Uncle Allen, who had worked at Duke University many years with "Dr. P." Once we realized that we had a common thread, our relationship took off running.

Like many others, "Dr. P" began to weaken with many health problems. Dementia began to be a part of "Dr. P's" life; however, his pleasant attitude and smile never left him. He was a blessing. Our bond continued, matter of fact, we became closer and closer. My last memory was when he returned from his daughter's house in San Francisco. It was "Dr. P's" last Christmas. I'm so glad he as able to make the trip and have one more good time! Thanks, "Dr. P" for blessing me so!

Mr. Bowman

When I reflect back on my times with Mr. Bowman, my first thought involves baths. In our first book, Octopus described the fear of the bath by dementia people because of the unknown and how important it is for the caregiver to take these fears away from these special people through trust and love. This is not the case. There are some people who just do not like baths period. This is the case of one Mr. Bowman.

Mr. Bowman was a very successful businessman, and although he had dementia, it had nothing to do with the fact that he hated baths—he absolutely hated them! During this part of my career, every one in our nursing community practically gave up on giving him a bath. He thus became my project. And, he was a project. I suspect that Mr. Bowman didn't all of a sudden hate baths. I believe he hated them a long time ago too.

I had a plan. Saturday nights would be instrumental in my attack; at least, I hoped so. I would experiment with "Therapeautic Fibbing." That is even if it weren't Saturday night we would make believe that it was. I knew that was the night of the weekly bath and probably, Mr. Bowman years ago gave his mother a fit, but eventually he gave in and took his bath. It was mandatory, so that was my plan. As a whole, the plan worked pretty well, but there were times when he needed more of a reason for a bath than just Saturday night.

As the Saturday night plan got old, I turned to perhaps the best plan. This same gentleman loved basketball and even though he was in Healthcare, I took him with the independent residents on the bus to the games with me. He loved this. He looked forward to having a big coke and a box of popcorn about as much as the game. This was the answer. When there was a game, that day became bath day. Although he still hated baths, this was a much better reason to take a bath than just being Saturday night!

My second thought of Mr. Bowman is taking him to the Davidson College basketball games, as you might have guessed. The story I'm about to tell will be a memory that will never leave me!

"We Damn Near Didn't Make It"

What words you must be thinking! And, what on earth could one be talking about? In our first book we acknowledged that going to the bathroom was a vital and necessary activity for all of us. Sometimes it is much easier than other times, but very necessary. Sometimes we have extreme difficulty and need special assistance or should I say, a beverage, such a grape juice as was the case with Mr. J. Then sometimes, as Brother Drum, and the rest of us know, we do not make it; and then, there are the times we do make it, but just barely. It is the later that this story will focus on.

The setting is the Belk Arena. The event is a college basketball game and as we later experienced there were more than one game going on. We also became aware there were more participants in the Belk Arena than the basketball players. There was also Mr. Bowman and myself. As the seconds ticked down on the clock of an exciting overtime game, the clock was ticking down on us. We were past overtime. We had reached sudden death or should I say, sudden mess if one caregiver by the name of TURNIP did not haul it! And, now, you guessed it, Mr. Bowman, who loved to go to ballgames, but hated baths, was ready to do that necessary activity. I knew, that if I didn't really move fast that activity would occur in Mr. Bowman's wheelchair, surrounded by thousands of fans and in a matter of seconds, their disappointments of the Wildcats getting beat would turn to where that terrible smell is coming from. I only had time for one thought and that was, unlike most occasions on outings with Healthcare. I was unprepared. This was an independent living event, which I took Mr. Bowman, as well as a busload of independent residents. I had no gloves, towels, or anything so I flew with Mr. Bowman. The wheelchair, Mr. Bowman, and I were really moving. The glares from the fans didn't slow us down. We had no time to spare. And, as mentioned earlier, we did make it, but barely. You know, this was an experience I'll never forget and you know,

Mr. Bowman, as long as he lived he never forgot that night. Sometimes it's funny what we remember about people. A lot of times we don't remember important things about a person, but some crazy experience or time we shared together.

That is the way it was with Mr. Bowman. Every time he saw me, he would say, "Ole Man Turner, we damn near didn't make it." He said this as long as he lived, even at his weakest condition. You know, I'll never forget it either, and probably years later when I think of Mr. Bowman this will be what I remember most. I am so thankful that God allows me into a human being's world enough to be able to even share a moment like this. This kind of relationship is like a home. The participants feel safe, secure, special, and loved.

"The Voice of New England"

Did you ever hear a beautiful voice? Sometimes people's greatest gift is their voice. Many times a person's voice can be so refreshing. It can also be very comforting—so pleasing to the ear. Sometimes a voice can be so special and have a special tone that seems to be a part of a region of the country. That was the case with "The Voice of New England." She was from New England and what a representative and what a lady!

Although she was from New England, most of the years of adult life were spent in Davidson. She was quite a representative for the little town of Davidson too. She was a lady of principles. She also was one who stood up for what is right in this ole world. She was able to use her gift of voice to benefit the citizens of Davidson on many occasions. The most noted of these was probably her fiery speech that was instrumental in getting the funds needed for the town library on Concord Road. People to this day are still talking about that speech, which seemed to turn the tide at a meeting that seemed to be going nowhere. Although I was not in Davidson, at the time, to witness this eloquent speech, I could picture this lady turning the tide.

Like many others, "The Voice of New England" loved her nickname. What joy she brought me each time I had the pleasure of taking her on outings, as well as medical appointments. As time went on, the medical appointments increased and her life became full of strokes and dementia, however, the voice was still present with its richness and freshness, which she became famous for. Our relationship continued to grow. We became closer and closer. Her condition gave her a greater need for me: and, you know, I needed her too. Like many of these special people, "The Voice of New England" gave me purpose. Her responses of love showed me that this is truly God's world and that I am doing His will. I also realized that love received and given in any circumstance or condition is a precious thing. And, as if I needed to know, love really does make the world go round!

"The Voice of New England" was a real blessing to me. In the end, it was my voice that provided a special lady with comfort, reassurance, and yes, love. This special lady "The Voice of New England" who had provided so many blessings to people with her voice, including myself, was now tuning into a voice by a person called "TURNIP." No matter how weak she got, she still knew me by my voice. I believe we knew each other through our hearts too. My last memories of "The Voice of New England" involved many strolls around our beautiful retirement community. These moments together were just as wonderful as our earlier times together, because there was love—thanks, "The Voice of New England"!

"My Panty Hose Man"

I know you must be really wondering, who on earth is "My Panty Hose Man," and why on earth would I be so bold as to give someone such a nickname. One is probably also questioning my thought process. I thought TURNIP took a great quality of time and consideration before coming up with the perfect fit—a perfect nickname. What happened with this one?

For those of you who don't know me as well as The Pines residents, in my first life I was a 3rd generation hosiery manufacturer of a family owned business. Having said that, "My Panty Hose Man," was a part of my first life. "My Panty Hose Man, like me, was involved in the hosiery business in a big way. Although he performed his career in High Point, there were times through the years that we crossed paths. At one time, the hosiery industry was an industry in which the various companies seemed to share secrets with each other for the betterment of the whole industry. So, on occasion, I was benefited greatly by "My Panty Hose Man" who shared with me his great experience and expertise. Like others, "My Panty Hose Man" came to The Pines. Our earlier friendship was rekindled. What a built-in bond we shared.

As time went on, "My Panty Hose Man" began to weaken both physically and mentally, however, we remained very close. He remained the gentleman who I knew in the hosiery business. His sense of humor was present too; however, it was the bond of the hosiery business that kept our conversations lively and continued to be our focal point. Once a panty hose man, and once "My Panty Hose Man," always "My Panty Hose Man"—thanks be to God!

"Good Doctor D."

"Good Doctor D." was a wonderful man with great intelligence. He was a gentleman and at the same time, which I learned during his weak moments, a strong man. His greatest gift, however, was his sense of humor. What wit!

Although, like other residents, he was very fond of his nickname, it was in his weakest moments that we became close. In his earlier days at The Pines, even though he should have had me drive him to medical appointments, he was independent and continued to drive, to the fear of all of us. As he weakened and dementia became a part of him, he asked me for help. As I responded to more wishes of this wonderful man, who had been a Davidson College Professor, our bond became stronger and stronger. Even as he got weaker and weaker, his personality which I dearly loved remained intact, especially his humor. Many times he would tell the nurses that he was trying to straighten TURNIP out, but he believed it would require more than prayer. What a sense of humor!

Fittingly, our last time together, his sense of humor was at its finest hour. I was taking "Good Doctor D." to the hospital, the day before he died, and we were traveling by the famous eating establishment "The Buttery and the Beanery" when I asked "Good Doctor D." if he had ever eaten there, and he replied, "I ate there once just so I could say I had done it"—what insight and humor. Thanks, "Good Doctor D.", for blessing me with your special humor!

"My Special Statesville Girl"

I know you are probably thinking, TURNIP has a lot of Statesville girls. And he does, but I've given them other nicknames. There has not been but one "My Statesville Girl"!

What a lady! Like many of my other Statesville girls, I was blessed by this special lady all of my life. Matter of fact, I grew up with her youngest daughter going to the same school and church. One of my blessings from being at The Pines is the fact that many relationships from the past are rekindled. The difference now is that I am now trying to take care of these special people who, at one time in my life, took care of me; and took me places. What a reversal! This was the case with "My Special Statesville Girl." It was now my turn to make her feel safe, secure, and special, just as she did for me as a little boy growing up. It was my time to give her joy, hope, and most important, love, especially as her condition weakened and time marched on.

As with the other residents, in order to be able to provide each person with joy, hope, and love, one needs to know as much about the person as possible. One must then be able to love that person no matter "What Condition their Condition is In" and you must have the want to. If you do what God wants you to do, all of these ingredients will be present. I know God is directing me. Now back to "My Special Statesville Girl." I had a head start with knowing her because of our past together, so I had plenty to work with.

Speaking of this, "My Special Statesville Girl" was so special that she provided me with many things to work with. She was a beautiful lady, who liked to dress up in fine clothes. She also liked to go out to parties, concerts, theater, and the country club. I believe it's important to create an environment that is conducive for each person to still be the special person God created them to be. In some instances, as with this special lady, it requires one to take this individual places.

As time passed on, "My Special Statesville Girl's" life became one full of dementia. To complicate things, she had macular degeneration, however there was still hope, joy, and love out there—possibility always. Her family knew she liked fine clothes so they continued to let her have fine clothes. Even though her eyesight had diminished, fine clothes could be felt. I believe she knew if she was dressed for the occasion or not. Throughout most of her life I still took her to the theater, which was located where I felt I could take good care of her. She loved going even though her eyesight limited her. I also took her to concerts, which she enjoyed. All of these events she was a part of the trips into Charlotte on the bus with the independent residents. As mentioned earlier, she loved to go eat lunch at the club. I was able to take her on the Healthcare outings to River Run, which made her extremely happy. When she weakened to a point she was unable to ride the bus, I took her to River Run in the car with me. As far as she knew, the special lady had a date with TURNIP. I feel very blessed to have been her date. It was an honor for me, and one that I'll never forget.

Speaking of being blessed, the last time "My Special Statesville Girl" did the honors was the last time I saw her. I had just arrived at Lake Norman Hospital to get a lady on the 3rd floor and transport her back to The Pines when I heard a familiar voice, which happened to be a nurse at Lake Norman, but also worked PRN at The Pines. She didn't realize I came for somebody, but she thought I came to see "My Special Statesville Girl." She requested that I go see her and see if she knew me, as she didn't know her; so I told her, "She will know me"; and sure enough, "My Special Statesville Girl" lit up like a Christmas tree when she heard my voice—how humbling! I know though that I am in the right place and at the right time, and most important I'm in God's plan. Thanks to "My Special Statesville Girl"—I love you and always will!

"Nanny"

"Nanny" was a very interesting lady and a proud great grandmother to boot. Although she had experienced many strokes and was paralyzed on the left side of her body and was victimized by dementia, she was always smiling and a blessing to all. As a result of the many strokes, "Nanny" could not speak very clearly; however, she talked anyway and I loved her.

Just as I've mentioned many times, when dealing with dementia people, it's not important that she isn't making any sense and you are not making sense, together you are communicating and that's all that matters. "Nanny" was a very courageous person and always gave me a lift.

Although each time together with "Nanny" was special to me, whether taking her for ice cream or doctor appointments, my most memorable trip was the Grand Opening of the new Cannon School in Concord. "Nanny" had such a good time. She had great ties to Concord and she was even honored at the ceremony. I can still see her beaming. Her smile will always be with me and what a gift one can receive—thanks, "Nanny." What a blessing—thanks be to God!

"Miss Coke"

"Miss Coke" was an easy nickname to come up with. As you might have guessed, she loved to drink Cokes. She also loved cigarettes too, but I decided "Miss Coke" would be a better nickname in our dear ole medical world we live in.

With regard to the dear ole medical world, I've always been of the opinion if somebody is 80 or 90 years old, they should be able to have Cokes and cigarettes if they want them. I also believe they should be able to eat their favorite foods too! If they haven't gotten a balanced diet by now, what difference does it make? Oh, well, back to our subject, "Miss Coke."

Like "Nanny," "Miss Coke" was a very unique and interesting person. Although she had dementia, she was still real sharp. She was very friendly and talkative; however, you never knew what was going to come out of her mouth. Even when you knew what was coming, she would surprise you to death—sometimes nice words, and some unprintable; but, she was honest and a whole lot of fun.

As for "Miss Coke" and me, we got along just wonderful. Maybe we bonded because I never seemed to know what's coming out of my mouth either. Anyway, we were very close.

Speaking of close, I believe she was one of those rare residents that truly loved me for all the right reasons, as well as the wrong reasons, but she loved me. With each passing day, if I hadn't made my way down to Healthcare to give that hug and kiss to her, she would have her caregiver stroll her until she found me. She would hunt me down. The memory that will last forever in my mind is "Hell, Turner, are you going to give me a kiss or are you just going to stand and look at me?" I can still hear "Miss Coke" saying that with so much vigor and I believe some crazy kind of love for some kind of crazy man; but, it's times like this, that I know I wouldn't trade places with anyone. Thanks, "Miss Coke," I love you too!

"Queen B"

Yes, another Queen—I've been blessed by being surrounded by a few in my second life. "Queen B" was another special lady that deserved to be a Queen too!

Like "My Favorite Author" and "My Queen Call," my relationship with "Queen B" got closer and closer after her husband's death. Like my "Favorite Author" and "Queen Call," I transported "Queen B" to her husband's funeral at DCPC. From that point our relationship together stepped up. It was at her husband's funeral that I became aware of something that bonded us for life. Ever since I came to The Pines in 1992, and each time I saw "Queen B" and her husband I kept thinking I knew them in my first life, but I could never pinpoint it, until the funeral. It dawned on me that I knew them from being a camper at Camp Carolina in Brevard. What a time to realize this. With this revelation at the funeral, I began to cry. Just think of all of the fun and memories we could have shared together while her husband was living if only I would have known, but I didn't. Once "Queen B" knew that I was a 3-time camper at Camp Carolina, I was her boy from then on. We bonded and got closer and closer.

At the time of her husband's death, she was already a victim of strokes and dementia, but what a lady! She had so many interesting stories to tell. And like "Miss Book Circle," she loved going places, even in her weakened condition. Like "Miss Book Circle" she had lived in Davidson almost her entire adult life, so she knew everybody. We went to weddings, social gatherings at the church, and many activities at the college. Like "Miss Book Circle," I was her date. You know, I felt honored, even though she didn't have much to choose from—TURNIP or TURNIP, but I did feel honored. I know I was blessed to share so many memories with such a lovely lady who liked to call me Turner Turner. I know you are thinking why on earth would she call me Turner Turner? It came about shortly after the death of her husband and before our relationship began to take off; when somehow she asked somebody my name and she thought I was Turner Turner. She always said that no mother in her right mind would name someone Turner Turner.

Well, back to our special lady, "Queen B." I cherish all of the times together, even going to the doctor, which can still be fun as long as love and humor are present. Love is the greatest gift and can take down all barriers and somehow, even in a weakened condition, *Inner Peace* was the result with "Queen B" even in her last days; but, you know, I believe *Inner Peace* is always the result with my special people because there is love. I feel so blessed for God to have given me the precious gift of love. I only pray I will always be able to use my gift for His glory. Although these special people feel *Inner Peace,* I believe I receive the most. Thanks to all of these special people and thanks to "Queen B"—I love you and always will!

One last thing to tell about "Queen B." Our last trip together came the day before she died, as we went to see her doctor in Charlotte. Somehow on the trip home, after eating peppermint ice cream, which we both loved, I went by her home that she had lived in raising her children and living in Davidson. Sometimes we would ride by her house, but not all times. It's almost like God was driving, in order for one special lady "Queen B" to see her home one last time. We were driving home and as always she said, "I wish we could find that recipe for cinnamon buns, like the ones we ate at Camp Carolina." I remember them well. She laughed at me because with all my experiences at camp, all I remembered was the cinnamon buns—they were good! I know now "Queen B" has found the recipe by now and is eating them every day—save some for me!

"Queen Lenox"

Yes, another Queen—and what a remarkable lady! She had a contagious sense of humor that would have one laughing forever. She also had a laugh of her own that brought joy to all who heard it and would, at times, even bring the house down!

"Queen Lenox" and I had many wonderful memories together. Our relationship was kindled when she was in Independent Living. You couldn't help but love her—she was so friendly and so easy to love. We hit it off immediately. Her husband and the "Queen Lenox" went to many concerts with me. I also took them to the airport many times during holidays to visit with their daughters, who both lived in the Boston area. I got to know their whole family and I was blessed by each one of them; but "Queen Lenox" was so special and we were so close. She even called me first from the hospital when her husband died and I went and brought her back home—how humbling; I believe God has empowered me to do what I do. I only pray I can continue to hear God's cry and do His will.

Like many of the residents, as time goes on, one weakens and begins to have medical problems. "Queen Lenox's" problems seemed to have started with her bad falls. Over a period of time she broke both of her hips twice, but what spunk! She was still such a blessing. Doctors dearly loved her. Each appointment was quite an experience and before we left the doctor's office the whole staff would be laughing so hard they were crying! What a lady! As time marched on, "Queen Lenox's" condition weakened and dementia found its home in her; but, her humor never left or desire to keep living, and having fun and she continued to like to read and play bridge. She also continued to go with me to eat "Cherry Garcia" ice cream which we both dearly loved, and last, she still wanted to travel and travel she did!

Speaking of travel, although I have many wonderful memories of this special lady, the thing I will always remember will be our next to last time at the airport together. I believe this encounter made us famous at Charlotte International Airport for all of the right and wrong reasons; but, when love is present and trust, I feel like things are perfect in this world. I believe this was the case at the airport with "Queen Lenox" and me—I know we had God's blessing—here's the incredible story.

When I took "Queen Lenox" to the airport, little did I know what we had in store—no idea! After all, we had done this airport thing many times. Everything had gone as planned departing as well as arriving. Each trip was the same—"Queen Lenox" riding in the wheelchair and smiling while I was pushing her through the concourse to board the plane—no hitch, so we did not expect one this time.

This time as I rolled the Queen down the concourse to board the plane, "Queen Lenox" expressed the desire to go to the little girl's room. Although I rolled her in a wheelchair, I also was carrying her walker. She believed that she would be able to go to the bathroom with her walker; so I helped her up to the entrance, and I waited; and waited; and waited; and waited. The whole time I was so concerned about my Queen, then, all of a sudden a lady came out running toward me saying, "Are you TURNIP?" After nodding my head, she informed me that my special lady was on the pot and weakened and could not get up. "Queen Lenox" had informed this lady to find TURNIP that he could take care of her. Don't you know this lady was impressed? Probably not, she was probably wondering where on earth one could find a man like this and what on earth is The Pines all about? I bet the lady will never forget us though.

I was relieved that "Queen Lenox" was all right and needed me; however, my next thought was how on earth is TURNIP going to sneak in the *women's bathroom*? I had experience going in women's dressing rooms to help with the dressing of these special ladies, and I had been in bathrooms at hospitals and on buses with special ladies, but never in a woman's bathroom; and certainly not at an international airport—never! What on earth was I going to do? Then all of a sudden, just like a miracle, an airline stewardess I knew came to my rescue and proceeded straight to the little girl's room to inform everyone in the sound of her voice that a man would be in the women's bathroom. With the cue, I headed in finding "Queen Lenox" sitting on her throne and at her finest hour. When she saw me she said, "TURNIP, I knew you would come to my rescue and take care of me." In this weak moment, she was so happy and enjoying every moment together, even in the bathroom. As I started to take care of this special lady, some egotistical US Air supervisor ran up and informed us that this was not a proper thing to do and expressed her wishes in a great huff. My friend, the airline stewardess said, "Can you get her off the pot?" Enough said and out the door the supervisor flew. An airport policeman, whom through the years I had gotten to know, replaced her. His attitude was quite different from the supervisor. He thought this was the funniest thing he had ever witnessed, especially at the airport. Between "Queen Lenox" laughing and the policeman, you couldn't hear anything in the bathroom—he was laughing so loud and shaking all over! As I proceeded to help the Queen, our eyes met, each staring a hole through each other and we were both shaking our heads and I think we were both thinking that it doesn't get any better than this—what a moment! Finally I took care of "Queen Lenox" and we headed for the plane on the wheelchair. As we got to the entrance, I got her out of the wheelchair and she put her arms around me and stood on my feet and we headed for the seat—what a beginning for Christmas and what Spirit and one that I will never forget; but, the story is not over.

After seeing that the plane carrying "Queen Lenox" to Boston took off, the policeman came up to me and informed me that there were unisex bathrooms on every concourse. I certainly had no idea. Because of this great source of knowledge given to me by the policeman, most likely I will not be in any more ladies bathrooms at Charlotte International Airport or any airports for that matter, but, you know, I'm glad I didn't know about the unisex bathrooms, because I would have missed a story full of love that was made possible by trusting in God's love to do miraculous things between a very special lady and a caregiver, who because of this story knows why he is here. Thank you, God and "Queen Lenox"—I love you!

A story like this never grows old and never ends as I've found out. Since 9/11 it is not as easy to take some of my special people to the airport as it once was; however, the beautiful story of "Queen Lenox" and me has made things easier. I am now recognized as being the man who went in the women's bathroom. Recently, employees of the airport have recognized me and have given me a pass to go on the concourse with my special people, thus, saving me a trip into a long line to get the pass—thanks, to "Queen Lenox" and to God again—I feel so blessed!

So, what's in a name for you and me? When a family member is first told that their loved one has some form of dementia, their first reaction is of horror. They believe their loved one will cease to exist. It is not uncommon for a relative to say, "My sister died yesterday. She had Alzheimer's, but I really lost her a few years ago."

Why is this? Does the relative feel that this person has lost the ability to communicate? Maybe, in the customary way they think the connection is lost. Is it? Not in my experience. It is just different.

In the end, we all forget a face, a date, a place, but we never forget the name written on our hearts. We all speak the same language of love. Share your uniqueness with them. So call your father by name, call the name of your mother, your sister, your brother, your aunt, your uncle, your neighbor with Alzheimer's while you can.

May you be encouraged to get into their world and give them a moment and revel in their happiness? If so, perhaps we will realize that the Alzheimer's patient's soul and brain are still intact, even if their memory is in the past and they can have tranquility.

What's in a name, exclusively Alzheimer's? Although the name Alzheimer's will still be a humbling disease, it will not be nearly as dreaded and the name will not have as bad a ring to it. The outlook will be bright because there will be love.

Sometimes memories are just insignificant ripples on a pond. Other times, they're *etched on the heart.*

Love Notes

Love Notes

T·U·R·N·I·P

TRUST · UNDERSTANDING · RESPECT · NURTURED · INNER · PEACE